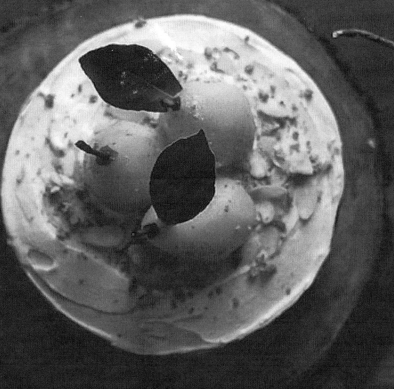

MACROSNUTRIENTS

MOST STRAIGHT FORWARD GUIDE TO UNDERSTANDING MACRONUTRIENTS AND FLEXIBLE DIETING/IIFYM

WILSON P.

Table of content

No table of contents entries found.

Introduction

The correct calorie and macronutrient intake effects the most important role in achieving high level physique goals. Tracking our total food intake is the easiest and most reliable way to lose body fat or gain lean body mass.

The main purpose behind guide is to help you better understand the relationship between how much and what we eat and the way our bodies look. My hope is that this information will save you a lot of time and effort as well. In the following chapters you'll learn how to estimate calorie needs for either fat loss or lean body mass gain. You'll also learn how to set your protein, fat and carb intake to best suit your goal.

If you'll understand this information, you'll be able to consume all sorts of delicious foods while losing fat or gaining muscle, you'll be free from dietary precepts and you'll be able to control your bodyweight and body composition however you want.

Chapter 1: Muscle and Strength

1. Total Amount of Calories consumed each day.

Nothing affects the way your body looks like as much as the total calories consumed do. Body fat is only burned when the body is in a caloric deficit.

2. Calories and macronutrients.

The protein, fat and carb ratio must be correctly set in order to prevent muscle loss or sustain muscle gain, a steady hormonal status and awesome exercise performance. In the next chapters you'll learn how to set up your calories and macronutrient numbers.

3. Fiber and Micronutrients as well.

Micronutrients have no direct effect fat loss and muscle growth (although sometimes they might do so through other mechanisms) but they are essential for health, recovery and good energy levels. For those exact reasons our diet must be highly nutritious. Fiber is important when cutting because it brings bulk to our diet helping with satiety and prevents constipation

4. Timing nutrition.

Nutrient timing refers to pre-workout nutrition, the number of meals you eat in a day, and how the food is distributed. It also refers to calorie and carb cycling as well. This is what you'd call the diet structure. Mainly for fat loss, the diet structure isn't that important as long as the calorie and macros needs are met. Although, the diet structure and food choices greatly influences whether you find it easy or hard to hit your numbers daily.

5. Supplementation.

Lastly the least important part overall are supplements. Most supplements are not that helpful but a lot of people place too much effort on them and lose focus of what matters most, calories and macros.I decided not to include a chapter on supplements in this mainly due to personally not using any and well experienced with them. Another reason is so that people convince themselves they don't require supplements in order to get great results. Refer to the nutrition pyramid below for a better understanding of the overall picture.

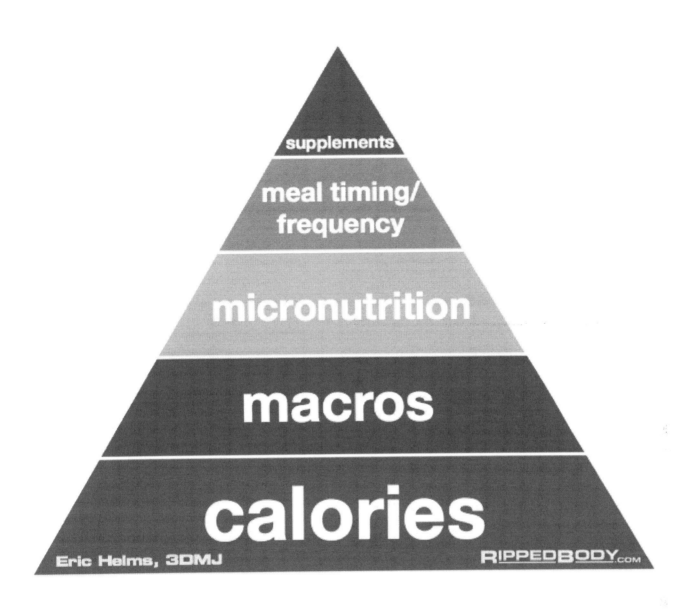

Chapter 2: The Importance of Calories

Since you decided to purchase this book, chances are you already know why calories are important and you only want to learn how to set your macros correctly. You'll read about that in the following chapters. For those of you who don't clearly understand the role of energy balance, we'll talk briefly about it here.

Calories are a measurement unit for energy. A calorie (kcal) is the amount of energy required to heat up one kilogram of water one degree Celsius. The energy our bodies burn and the potential energy in food is measured in calories.

All the foods we eat are loaded with calories. Any move we make (including our bodily organs own movement such as heart beats) burns calories. Depending on how much we consume and how much we move, three possible things can happen:

1. When we eat about as many calories as we burn. In this case our weight will stay the same.
Most people maintain this equilibrium unconsciously over long periods of time.

2. We eat more calories than we burn. We steadily start gaining weight. This calorie surplus can be transformed into fat and/or muscle. This will depend on how we train and if we do a lot of intensive exercise such as weightlifting.

3. We burn more calories than we eat. In this case, we will steadily start to lose weight. That calorie deficit forces the body to tap into its own fat reserves for energy. Depending on the
size of the deficit, how we train and the macronutrients we eat, the body will obtain the extra energy from burning fat and/or muscle. This is why a lot of people tend to go on Keto or low carb diets, so that your body will start to dip into the fats after all the carbs are burnt out.

Methods and Cause

For most people this concepts shouldn't be all that new. Even so, many people may not have
heard the role of energy balance explained properly in this way because most diet books skip this part entirely.

Most dietitians don't realize that people don't want to eat less, which kinda sucks. So they
came up with diet rules that make people eat less in an indirect way. Some popular
methods for weight loss include: low carbohydrate or fat intake, clean eating (or eliminating certain foods based on arbitrary reasons), eating only at certain times,

intermittent fasting and many more. It doesn't matter which method is heavily promoted its not that important because the cause of weight loss or weight gain is the same: total calorie intake

One important thing to note is that, no matter what type of diet you are on, it is still a calorie deficit. It doesn't matter if this is low carb, low fat, intermittent fasting, or Paleo. It's a way to restrict calories without overthinking it. Of course, a lot of diets come with health benefits as well, but it isn't the main reason why people are shedding off fat.

Tricking the Mind

This doesn't mean that the dietitians and nutritionist that offer their advices are intentionally trying to be bad about it. They know that any diet works as long as it creates a caloric deficit and they hope people will start eating less by following a specific set of direction. Most people would rather follow some simple direct rules, indirectly create a caloric deficit and get the process complete.

In order to better understand what I mean by indirect energy deficit, check out the list below and
you'll see an interesting pattern:

Do more cardio = burn more calories = energy deficit = weight loss
Eat only "clean foods" = eat fewer calories = energy deficit = weight loss
Don't eat carbs = eat fewer calories = energy deficit = weight loss
Don't eat after a certain eating window = eat fewer calories = energy deficit = weight loss
Consciously eat fewer calories = energy deficit = weight loss
All of the methods from that list work and can lead to fat loss.

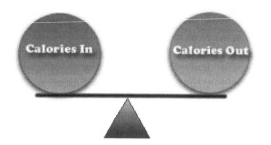

Weight Maintained
Isocaloric Balance
Energy In = Energy Out

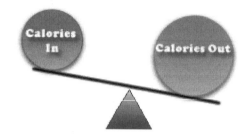

Weight Loss
Negative Caloric Balance
Energy In < Energy Out

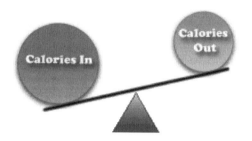

Weight Gain
Positive Caloric Balance
Energy In > Energy Out

Problems with calories restriction.

Personally, I'm not entirely against the method for restricting calories for weight loss but in my professional opinion every person with advanced physique goals should understand the actual cause of weight change. If they don't learn about the energy balance they risk confusing the method with the cause.

For instance, if a person believes eating clean is the cause of fat loss they will not understand why it's possible to hit a plateau. When their weight stalls they'll have no idea why and won't know how to adjust things. When a person eats low-fat type of diets, they'll also be in risk with a lot of other health problems due to the fact that our body actually *needs fats.* That is why if you're on a low-fat diet, you should go for healthy fats such as almonds, olive oil and more.

This is a similar song and dance for people who do cardio for fat loss. They should know in advance that exercise in and of itself is not the cause for fat loss but it's actually a method for creating an energy deficit.

Calories for weight gain.

We've mostly talked about fat loss but the total energy intake is just as important for gaining weight. Muscle growth depends to a large extent on a calorie surplus and on weight gain. An energy surplus means eating more calories than our body burns at our current weight and activity level.

Goals

When people comment about how they'd like to gain weight, my thought goes straight to them wanting to gain muscle not body fat. Unlike fat gain, muscle gain is slow and it doesn't usually require a heavy calorie surplus. Overeating too much over maintenance will exceed the amount of nutrients the body uses for creating muscle tissue and the rest will be turned into fat. For this reason, setting a calorie surplus correctly is the most important factor for gaining muscle with little to no fat gain.

Now, when people comment how they'd like to lose weight I assume they want to lose fat not muscle. In order to achieve this effect one should also pay strict attention to the macronutrient composition of their diet not just calories. Losing body weight doesn't ensure that your body composition (ratio between fat and muscle) is getting better. Furthermore, they should not lose body weight too fast as this usually leads to muscle catabolism and strength loss as well.

For this upcoming chapter you'll learn how to properly set a calorie deficit for weight loss or a
calorie surplus for gaining lean body mass. But before that let's address a topic that's
sometimes confusing for most: the difference between calories, nutrients and food.

Chapter 3: Nutritional foods and calories

For this part of the chapter we'll talk about the difference between the intake of calories, nutrients and food. Some of you may find this to be very basic information, so go ahead and skip it. For those of you who aren't interested in fitness or bodybuilding don't think about their daily calorie or macronutrient intake, they simply think about how much food they eat. And as we know, the number of calories and nutrients contained in a certain amount of food can vary drastically depending on the food choices.

Calories

As was previously mentioned before, a calorie (kcal) is a measurement unit for energy
and is equal to the amount it takes to heat up one kilogram of water one degree Celsius.
When estimating a person's energy requirement we're estimating how many calories
that person needs to function the way they do now. And when we're saying a food has X
amount of calories we refer to how much potential energy is contained in that food.

Macronutrients

There's around three macronutrients that form the basis of all foods: protein, fats and carbohydrates. A fourth macronutrient would be alcohol but as im sure you're aware, this isn't normally found in most foods.
Each macronutrient contains a certain energy value:

1g of protein = 4 kcal
1g of carbs = 4 kcal
1g of fats = 9 kcal
1g of alcohol = 7 kcal

For most areas of the world, the energy value of a food is measured for 100g of product. That
means the energy value of a food is determined by the macronutrients it contains in 100g. Most people tend to leave out alcohol when it comes to counting macros.

For Instance: 100g of whole wheat bread contains the following macronutrients - 9g
protein, 3g fats, and about 50g of carbs. The energy contained in 100g of bread would
therefore be: 9g protein x 4 kcal + 3g fats x 9 kcal + 50g carbs x 4 kcal = 263 kcal.

I'm sure most people reading this already know this information but it's always good to have a refresher on the basics.

In the upcoming chapter we'll discuss about each macronutrient in more detail because they affect the body differently and each one is important. The distinction between total calorie intake
and macronutrient intake becomes important when we talk about body composition and not just body weight. Two people can consume similar amounts of calorie but depending on the macronutrients those calories comes from they can get very different results in their body composition.

Foods

Clearly people consume foods and not calories and macros. And foods will vary greatly in their macronutrient and calorie content. The foods we consume to reach our macros are important for satiety, health and vitality.

For instance you can eat 100g of carbs from potatoes or low-fat cookies. Although the energy you'd get would be the same (400kcal), you must eat 500g of potatoes compared to only 140g of cookies. It's obvious that from a satiety point of view it would be much wiser to choose the potatoes over the cookies.

Food Quantity and Energy Value.

The average person only thinks about how much food they're consuming and not about the
calories or macronutrients obtained from that amount of food For this reason a lot of people Complain about not losing weight even though they're eating very little. These people only eat very little but because of their food choice makes their calorie intake is
actually pretty high.

Here's an example, if a girl goes out and gets a small Mochaccino and two cookies (0.4 oz. each)
That's a 325 kcal "meal". She ate almost nothing but has already used about one quarter of the calories she needs to eat to stay in a deficit.

The same girl could instead have one cup of cottage cheese (225g) with berries and feel much more satisfied for the same number of calories. Furthermore, the higher protein content of this food would probably support her physique goals better than the refined carbs.

Recent research shows that the source of macronutrients does not influence body composition. That means as long as you hit your macros you can eat more or less whatever you want and achieve your physique goals.

Although, eating only processed foods can lead to micronutrient deficiencies and health problems in the long run. Also our food choices greatly affect how satiating our meals are and how sustainable our diet is.

Low calorie foods such as lean meats, vegetables, fruits and root vegetables would allow us to eat a large quantity of food for minimal calories. This helps stave off hunger and cravings which makes it much easier for us to remain in a caloric deficit.
Additionally, whole foods would provide more micronutrients (vitamins & minerals) and fibre which will support our health and vitality.

Chapter 4: Energy Expenditure

Estimating the Total Energy Expenditure is considered the most important part when it comes to creating an efficient diet plan. Once you become aware how many calories you burn at your current weight and daily activities, then you can adjust that number up or down for lean bulking or cutting.

There are a tons of formulas out there that give you a decent estimation for the number of calories a person needs to eat at a given weight based on gender, age, height, and activity level.
For this chapter we'll journey through the most popular of these formulas, you'll learn their strengths and limitations and how to utilize them to determine your calorie needs.

Calorie Estimation.

A person's Total Energy Expenditure (TEE) is composed of:

1. BMR – Basal Metabolic Rate. BMR is the amount of energy expended while at rest in
a neutrally temperate environment, in the postabsorptive state (which means that the
digestive system is inactive, which requires about twelve hours of fasting). BMR includes the energy consumed by breathing, pumping blood, cellular growth and repair, and any other biological process necessary to maintain life.

2. TEA – Thermic effect of activity. TEA is the amount of energy expended through all
voluntary and involuntary movements. The voluntary movements would be things such as
lifting weights, cardio, walking to work, and so forth. The involuntary movements are the
movements we perform unconsciously such as changing position while sitting, bumping our leg on the floor, tapping the table and more. These unconscious

movements have been named NEAT (Non-exercise activity thermogenesis) and it seems they vary substantially between people.

3. TEF – Thermic effect of food. TEF is the amount of energy expended for the digestion and absorption of food (yeah ingesting calories burns calories). TEF is not equal for all foods. Alcohol (20%) and protein (20-35%) require the most energy for digestion. Carbs stored as glycogen require about 5-6% of the total calories, carbs converted to fat use up to 20% of the total calories and most fats can be absorbed with almost no energy cost (2-3%). Overall TEF amounts to about 10-15% of TEE (but the
formulas below already take it into account when calculating BMR).

So in order to find your maintenance calories we need to include BMR along with TEA.

Basal Metabolic Rate estimation.

One of if not THE most popular formula for calculating BMR is the Harris-Benedict equation.
This is a fantastic measurement for the general population. Here are some examples of this on how this all works out:

The Harris-Benedict Equation

Men: 66 + (13.75 x weight in kilograms) + (5 x height in cm) - (6.76 x age in years) =
BMR
Women: 655 + (9.56 x weight in kilograms) + (1.85 x height in cm) – (4.68 x age in years) = BMR

Another great equation for calculating BMR is the Katch-McArdle equation. It works great for lean athletic people because it takes into account Lean Body Mass (LBM). Fat mass does not require much energy to maintain but muscle mass does. A 180lb male at 8% body fat will have a significantly higher BMR compared to a 180lb male at 20% body fat.

People who use this equation need to be completely honest about it. The majority of people tends to underestimate how much fat they have by 2-3%. I've actually had clients who thought they their body fat was half of what it actually was. If you don't really know your body fat percentage check the formula below.

The Katch-McArdle Formula

Men & Women: 370 + (21.6 x LBM in kilograms) = BMR
Another amazing equation i discovered a while back that works great is called Mifflin-St Jeor. Keep in mind that this does not count LBM in but works very effectively.

The Mifflin-St Jeor Formula

Men: (10 x weight in kg) + (6.25 x height in cm) – (5 x age in years) + 5 = BMR

Women: (10 x weight in kg) + (6.25 x height in cm) – (5 x age in years) – 161 = BMR

I pretty much got the same result with both the Katch-McArdle and the Mifflin-St Jeor so it's really up to you as the reader on which you wish to use.

Chapter 5: Calorie Deficit

Now that you've learned how to maintenance calories in order to lose weight it's time to set a caloric deficit.

There only one person we can go to who found the key to all of this and that's Strasser et al who actually proved that fat loss depends on energy deficit only, independent of the method used to create it. For this study, two groups of people were put into an energy deficit but through different methods: one group increased their energy expenditure through cardio while eating the same way and the other one did no cardio but ate fewer calories. The conclusion of the study both groups showed the same weight reduction.

So there are three ways to create an energy deficit: increase total physical activity, eat less or do a bit of both at the same time.

The best fat loss results are usually seen with a moderate calorie deficit. This allows for steady fat loss while also preserving lean muscle mass. Ideally you'd use a deficit of about 20-25%. For most people this would mean 500-700 kcal under maintenance.

Calorie Deficit of 25%

With a 25% energy deficit most people will lose somewhere around 1-1.5 lbs (500-700g) of fat per week. Overweight folks will usually lose more than that, about 1.5-2 lbs (700g-1kg) per week.

Guys who are very lean themselves (9% body fat or less) should use a slightly lower deficit (15-20%) or cycle calories. Because they have less fat overall, the risk of muscle and/or strength loss is increased when using a larger deficit.

Adjustments will most likely need to be made for these numbers as you're losing body fat and weight. If you no longer lose weight at the rate of 1-1.5 lbs per week, lower your calorie intake by 8-10%. If you find you're losing weight too fast, increase your calories by 5-10%.

Setting the deficit properly

A great calorie deficit restricts the necessary amount of energy to force the human body to burn body fat, but not enough to interfere with muscle recovery and growth.

consuming much less than your body burns, will lead to a much rapid drop in fat, but the huge
calorie deficit will also lead to muscle loss, hormonal imbalances and decreased physical
performance. Totally not worth it to be honest. On the other hand, if you eat too close to maintenance, fat loss will be too slow and you'll lose time and motivation.

The most ideal calorie deficit would be about 20-25% under maintenance because it produces fast fat loss without negative effects on lean body mass and performance.

Chapter 6: The Calorie Surplus

Muscle growth is maximized only when consuming large amounts of calories than we burn. New
muscle tissue cannot be created out of nothing; therefore a slight surplus of calories is necessary for furthering growth.

The amount of nutrients our bodies require to develop new muscle tissue every day is believe or not really low. This is the reason why only a few hundred calories over maintenance are enough to maximize lean muscle growth.

Plenty of people make the unfortunate mistake of consuming far too much during a bulking phase and end up gaining more fat than muscle. More often than not these guys look worse at the end of the bulk than when they started.

My personal belief on this is for us to strive for lean gains as much as we can while not compromising the rate at which we can gain muscle and strength. A significant amount of fat gain should be allowed otherwise our progress would be significantly slower.

Chapter 7: Known people behind weight change

After a couple of weeks into cutting, some folks have reported reaching a plateau when they no longer lose fat eating the same way as before. No worries though, this is completely normal. The first reason has to do because they're lighter than previously before. Remember from the last chapter we spoke about the Total Energy Expenditure and what it's composed of.

If you remember from before you'll start to notice the total energy expended by all three consumers changes along with weight and food intake.

When you begin to consume food at a deficit TEF goes down simply because we eat less. BMR also goes down because we're lighter. TEA goes down as well because a smaller body burns less energy during any activity.

Something else that everyone will find incredibly interesting is that NEAT usually drops too. One of the ways our body tries to conserve energy during a deficit is by reducing spontaneous, unnecessary movements. This adaptation is more pronounced in some people than others but those who are low NEAT responders usually report feeling lethargic during a caloric deficit. IF we move less, we're going to burn less energy.

Changes in Hormones.

I'm sure most of you readers are aware of the hormone called Leptin. For those who don't, Leptin is a master hormone involved in maintaining our metabolic rate and also controls hunger to a large extent.

The amount of leptin a person holds all depends on our fat mass and our food intake. Reducing our calories and we start losing fat, leptin automatically lowers causing a series
of adaptations: our metabolic rate is slightly reduced, hunger is increased, testosterone levels decrease, and NEAT goes down.

An interesting tidbit to note down is that the drop in metabolic rate is not linear. A slight decrease in calorie intake and fat mass produces a larger decrease in metabolic rate than normally
expected. So at the beginning of the diet we see a significant drop but then our metabolic rate remains relatively stable decreasing slowly as we lose more body fat.

This finally explains why the deficit we've initially set no longer works after a couple of weeks.

Our lighter bodies utilize less energy overall, we consume less food and our metabolic rate has probably slowed down by 10-15%.

The solution for this?

When the weight begins to stall we are going to reduce our calorie intake again or increase
our energy expenditure. My personal recommendation is to reduce the calorie intake by 8-10%, increasing expenditure by 8-10% or do both at the same time really it all comes down to what you prefer to do.

Some folks have even discussed about "the starvation mode" and how it's a mistake to create a calorie deficit again after reaching the plateau. Well what other options are available to us? In order to lose fat we must be at a deficit.

No research performed has ever shown that a person's metabolism can slow down so much that it will make it impossible to lose any body fat. So when someone says they are not losing fat because they're eating too little, it's best to ignore them.

Weight Stalled even after consuming large amounts of calories.

Even so, it's possible to have a large to moderate deficit and still not lose weight due to water retention. Dieting, training and mental stress is main factor to increase cortisol levels which normally lead to water retention.

This doesn't mean fat isn't being lost. The reduction in fat mass may be masked by the lack of weight change and increased subcutaneous water. After a couple of days have passed the water should be flushed out and we'll see the reduction in weight and fat.

Influences behind weight gain.

The human metabolism protects itself against weight loss much more than it does against weight gain. This makes a lot sense from an evolutionary point of view because only in our modern society has fat gain become a recent health problem. We do have some mechanisms for preventing weight gain but they seem to be more evolved for some people better than others. An ideal calorie surplus can only be set through performed experiments. With a surplus of 200- 300kcal some people gain muscle and strength ideally while others don't receive any growth. Why could that possibly be? The surplus we set on paper is often very different from the actual surplus that occurs.

As soon a consumption of food begins, TEF goes up. More food means more energy is required to digest and absorb it. BMR and TEA also go up because a larger body burns more calories
both at rest and during activity.

Although the largest difference comes down to Non-Exercise Activity Thermogenesis or NEAT for short. When we consume more, our body usually tries to protect against weight gain by increasing our spontaneous and unconscious movements to burn energy. This is exactly the
opposite of what occurs during a fat loss phase.

Adjusting Calories when attempting to lean bulk.

Mey personal suggesting for you dear readers is to begin with only 200-300 kcal over maintenance and see if any gains are reached.If you gain too slowly, then increase the calories as needed. Remember to make small increases in calories. This way you'll avoid unnecessary fat gain.

Chapter 8: Macronutrients Placement

Once you've adjusted the calories correctly for either a cut or a bulk, the next step is to determine from which macronutrients those calories are going to come from. For those who want fantastic results remember that it's not enough only to count calories. Each macronutrient has it's own role and should never be ignored.

When it comes to a cut, a good ratio of macros will help maintain or increase muscle mass and performance, support healthy hormone levels and help with satiety. Furthermore, beginners almost always gain muscle mass during a cut if they're careful to hit their macros.

When bulking up, a high intake of protein and carbs will support muscle growth and recovery
while also providing the necessary energy to push yourself in the gym. Getting your macros
mostly from whole foods will also help with satiety - preventing overeating and fat gain.

Protein.

The most essential macronutrient in any diet is protein, that's why we'll discuss it first.
Decent amount of protein intake plays a major role in the maintenance of muscle mass while
in a caloric deficit. When losing weight, the body loses more amino-acids that it retains
and for that reason you must eat more dietary protein.

Research has shown that 1-1.4 grams of protein per lb of body weight (2.2-3g per kg) is ideal for
fat loss.
So a 165 lbs male would eat about 165g of protein a day. A guy weighing 176 would eat
about 175-180g of protein a day.

This formula cannot be applied for those significantly overweight. Protein is important for the

maintenance of lean mass but in their case a big part of their body weight is fat. For them
Its personally recommended that a smaller intake of protein, about 0.8g per lb of BW. So a 220 lbs guy would eat 220 x 0.8 = 175g of protein a day. When he gets to a lower body fat level, he can
increase their protein intake.

With maintenance or a lean gaining phase protein does not need to be as high as during a deficit. There is still however a protein threshold that needs to be met in order to maximize protein synthesis.

Body Fats.

Fats are incredibly important for body fats. A diet too low on fats leads to hormonal imbalance,
including testosterone production. On the other hand, a high fat diet does not support muscle growth and strength and is also bad for satiety due to fats being the most nutrient dense nutrient. Because of this it's recommend you set fat intake at 25% of total calories, regardless if it's for a bulk, cut or maintenance. This moderate intake is plenty enough to stimulate anabolic hormone release and also leaves plenty of room for carbs.

Carbs

The other half of calories will come from carbohydrates which will be the main key piece of macronutrient on this diet. This is mainly because carbohydrates support recovery and high intensity muscular work. Think of carbs as fuel for high intensity anaerobic workouts.

Carbs also support leptin, the hormone that regulates appetite and metabolism. High amounts of carbs support the testosterone to cortisol ratio in active individuals, leading to better
hormonal profile. They will also keep the stomach satisfied and promote relaxation and better quality of sleep (its been show that some people can't sleep due to low amounts of carbs).

To calculate carbs multiply grams of protein by 4 and grams of fat by 9 and then add these two numbers together. Next, subtract this number from total calories. Take that number and divide it by 4 to get grams of carbs per day.

Learning to Count Macros.

For this part we shall be using kinobody rules for counting macros:

First Rule: Keeping it simple.

Most of you will want to keep your diet as simple and effortless as possible. For this very reason I personally recommend using simplified rules. The following include:

1. Don't waste time counting calories from low amounts of fibrous leafy greens.

Believe me on this, there is nothing to gain from becoming completely obsessive and measuring every ounce of your vegetables. These foods are very high in vitamins/minerals/fiber and very low in calories. Remember that.

Personal recommendation for eating a moderate intake of fibrous vegetables with each meal without regard for calorie/macro intake.

If you're consuming more than 500g of vegetables per day then my personal recommendation for everyone is to lower your total energy intake by 100kcal so it will automatically cover the calories from vegetables. If you're eating even more than that then you should start counting calories from them too.

2. Don't waste time counting calories from low calorie condiments.

Low calorie sauces add barely any calories to a meal. Just keep in mind of how much you use and there is no need to have to count that towards your calorie/macro intake.

3. Stop wasting time counting trace proteins.

Starchy carbs usually contain trace amount of protein but this should definately be ignored.

It's simpler just to count your protein from meat. So a huge serving of potatoes will most likely contain 10g of protein. Consider that extra protein a bonus. When you begin to count protein from starches it makes things very complicated when you're increasing or decreasing your carb intake. Furthermore. you don't want to reduce any meat intake because you are consuming more starches. Meat intake should remain relatively constant.

4. Don't panic about not reaching the exact amount of calories and Macronutrients.

Try to get the best possible accuracy that you can. So within 5g of your fat intake, within 10g of protein and carb intake and within 50 calories of calorie intake. Trying to be completely accurate is not possible, and if you think you've achieved the perfect aim, then you're most likely wrong.

This is mainly due to food labels and measuring your food isn't even completely correct. You can't be 100% correct on this, you just need to be within the right line of sight.

Second Rule: Use an application.

In order to keep a record of everything you consume and so on it's recommended to use a helpful smart phone app. I personally use FatSecrets, it's a simple and easy to use app that has many useful functions. It allows for customization of your daily calories and macros, you can look up practically any food, scan barcodes, develop custom foods, and even track your weight and measurements.

The customized food function is incredibly useful. It allow people to find out how many carbs are in a serving of potatoes, rice, rice pasta and allows customization of food subtracting the trace
protein and trace protein calories. This way it won't count the trace nutrients towards the
calorie and macro count.

Third Rule: Electronic Food Scale.

Electronic food scale are incredibly useful tools to keep around the house. This allows anyone to quickly and seamlessly weigh their food so they can accurately enter it into the app to determine the number of calories and macros being consumed..

Fourth Rule: Raw meat should be weighed.

Lots of people tend to be confused on whether they should weigh the meat before or after cooking.

For the best results you should weigh it in the raw state. Although, you need to make sure that you are using the uncooked nutrition information when you enter it into the application.
The main reason is cause cooking your meat can reduce the weight of the food by 25-35%. So if you are weighing your chicken raw and entering it into your app as grilled chicken your calorie and protein numbers will be much higher than they should.

Normally, a grocery store bought meats the nutritional information is listed on the back. This refers to it in it's raw state. Go by those measurements. 100g of raw meat most likely has around 20g of protein. Depending on the type of meat, there could be anywhere from 0-20g of fat. These fat numbers need to be counted towards your macro and calorie intake.

If it Fits your Macros.

Sometime around 2009-2010 the idea that anyone can eat anything they want on a cut without compromising their results started to gain popularity on the bodybuilding.com forum.

With this being a new spanking ideas, loads of people started asking if they can eat pizza, chips, bananas,chocolates and so on. At first people took the time to write long answers to each comment explaining that they could eat whatever they wanted as long as it could fit in their macros. But over time people continued to ask the same thing, over and over. To keep it short they used the pharse:

"IIFYM"

Then everyone started using this acronym to answer those types of questions. Shortly after, IIFYM became a huge deal for people all over the world.

What is IIFYM?

IIFYM stands for if it fits your macros. Some people like to call if flexible dieting. Traditionally losing weight meant calorie tracking. Getting in fewer calories than what you are putting out means that you will lose weight over time. Eat more than what your maintenance calorie is and that means that you'll gain weight. That type of diet might not work for everyone.

IIFYM eliminates the calorie tracking perspective, instead, you'll be tracking your "macros". As long as you hit certain numbers, there's theoretically no limitation on what foods you can use to meet them. This is why it is called flexible dieting because of the fact that there are no food restrictions. This is however not necessary a good thing. We'll go over why this might not be the best option later in this article.

To make IIFYM work, you have to understand the principal of key nutrients or things can go terribly wrong, but if you have a good understanding of macro and micro nutrients, then IIFYM can be an extremely flexible diet that you can actually stick to.

Macros, short for "macronutrients," is the term used to describe the three major (or macro) nutrients: protein, carbohydrates, and fat. One of the biggest problems with traditional calorie tracking is that it's hard to stick to. With macros, it's more about eating a more well-balanced diet because if done right your macros shouldn't lead you to eat a bunch of junk food that isn't good for your body.

For example, let's take a look at a sample macronutrient of a chocolate cake. According to FatSecrets, a chocolate cake with chocolate frosting contains 34grams of carbs, 10g of fats, and 2g of protein (rough estimate). If you eat 3 pieces of chocolate cake, you'll be getting in approx. 103g of carbs, 30g of fats, and 6g of protein. Obviously, we all know that eating chocolate cake isn't the healthiest option. If you know that your daily macros cannot exceed 150 carbs, then you might stay away from any more cakes for the rest of the day. This is a good way to keep your foods and nutrients in check. At the same time, you won't go over your limits because you will be spending your other macros on protein for the rest of the day instead.

The good thing about IIFYM is that there is no restrictions or elimination of food groups, which means it is a diet that is sustainable. Another good thing about IIFYM, unlike fasting, is that there isn't a certain time window of the day on when you can eat and when you cannot eat. This diet believes that your stomach doesn't necessary have a clock or timer, as long as it fits your macros.

If performed correctly IIFYM will help you roll through your day with a good amount of energy and body balance.

Here are some benefits of being on IIFYM:

No restrictions or limits – As mentioned above, there are no restrictions or elimination making this diet much more sustainable in the long run.

Perfect for the social world – One of the hardest problems with going on another diet is that most diets tend to eliminate food groups or food types. For example, low carb diets like keto will fully eliminate carbs. Even though there are a lot of restaurants that offer low carb options, it can still be a hassle to get out of your way just to eat with a friend. Following an IIFYM approach promotes less stress in these sorts of situations. You can just eat more or less of a certain macro than planned at an earlier meal.

Performance – Due to the fact that IIFYM is a really well balanced diet, you should be able to up your performance and energy levels because you are having enough proper nutrients to help your body make it through the day.

Doing IIFYM the correct way

Sames as anything else in this world of ours some people take IIFYM to the extreme and eat only protein shakes, fast food and sweets because it fits in their macros. While yes strictly for body composition it makes no difference, it does lack vitamins, minerals and fibre can lead to health problems in the future. Furthermore, packaged food usually contains unhealthy amounts of fats, preservatives and other chemicals which can cause problems when eaten in massive amounts.

The main point to making IIFYM work fantastically is to get the majority of your calories (80-90%) from whole foods and the rest from whatever you want.

The downsides and pitfalls of IIFYM

No diet is perfect and there's always a downside to everything. One of the reasons why IIFYM receives a lot of rants is because a lot of people aren't approaching IIFYM correctly. This has given the approach a reputation as being unhealthy, even though it shouldn't be.

One of the downsides to IIFYM is that it is *too flexible*. This leads to a lot of people eating a bunch of junk as a part of their daily diet. Most people don't understand the difference between good carbs and bad carbs. Because of this reason, they think they can consume any food and still hit their macros. The problem with this is that if you are not eating nutrient dense foods, you will end up feeling more hungry and you won't get enough nutrients to allow your body to function correctly.

The second downside and pitfall to IIFYM are that most people on this diet miss out on their micronutrients. Macronutrients are the carbs, protein, and fats, whereas micronutrients are the essential vitamins and minerals. They play crucial roles in your training and recovery. Beginners tend to reach for cookies to hit their carb macros over something more nutrient dense like broccoli or asparagus. Fortunately, this is an easy problem to fix. Make sure you choose healthier options when it comes to hitting your macros. Opt for veggies over cookies, opt for fruits over ice cream etc. In conclusion, to make IIFYM work at it's best to choose healthier alternatives to hit your macros with.

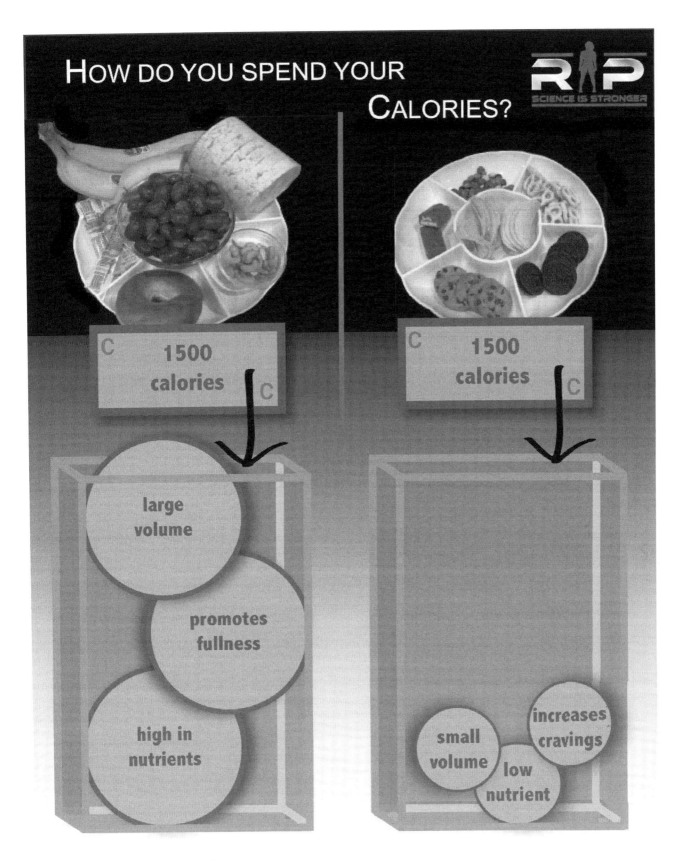

Finding your IIFYM split

Once you figured out your ideal daily calorie intake, you will need to choose a split. This varies depending on the end goal. The general rule of thumb is:

Bodybuilding – 40% protein / 40% carbs / 20% fat

Performance – 50% carbs / 30% protein / 20% fat

Lose weight – 40% protein / 30% carbs / 30% fat

You would take the ideal calorie number that you generated above and split it accordingly based on the split that you choose to go with.

There is no "wrong" macro split. It will ultimately come down to what you feel most comfortable with and can maintain. As long as you're in a caloric surplus or deficit, you should progress in the right direction. Your split will make a difference in how you feel and perform along the way, and in how fast you get where you want to go.

Apps that help with tracking your macros

Of course, you can always just write down everything, but that would be a pain. Luckily we have technology nowadays that can help you with keeping track of everything. Some of my favorite apps include the following:

FatSecrets – This is my most favorite app when it comes to tracking macro and calories. It is extremely useful friendly and they have a tab specifically made for macros so you can see your progress. It will even notify you if you went over your macros for the day.

MyFitnessPal – Most fitness and bodybuilders live by this app. It was one of the early adapters in the fitness space. There are a few things that I don't like about this app. First, a lot of the data are inaccurate. There are a lot of user generated data, making it difficult to know which ones are correct and which ones are not. The second thing that I don't like is that there are a lot of display advertising which I'm not a huge fan of.

Loseit! – This is a rather new app that I discovered which allows you to take a picture of a photo and the app will try its best to guess what food it is. I gave it a try and while it's an awesome app, I liked Fatsecrets a lot more.

There are a lot of other apps out there. If you come across one that you think it's good, please let me know by commenting below!

Should my macros stay the same every day?

This is fully up to you. Personally, I like to change my macros depending on my goals and my performance that day. I like to keep the carbs lower and protein higher on my rest days, while increasing my carbs on my workout days. The thing about dieting is that there isn't a single method that works for everyone. We can only follow certain rules of thumb, but at the end of the day, you have to figure out what works best for your body.

Simple ways to create a meal plan

If you don't want to bother add all that information consistently into an application, the alternative is to use a meal plan. After creating hundreds of meal plans for myself and for clients I've finally found a very efficient way to do it. If you're somebody that doesn't have time, then I would recommend that you use a meal planning service like this - http://nutritionhacks.io But, here is step by step guide on how you can get started on your own

1. Preferred meal frequency and food distribution

As long as you're ensuring total macronutrient intake for the day is optimal, how the diet is structured isn't that much important. Studies have shown that small and frequent meals do not speed up the metabolism, eating a large meal in the evening doesn't make you fat, you don't need to eat protein every 3 hours and you can skip a meal or two without going catabolic.

Now what this really means is that you can have as many meals as possibly want along with choosing at each time of the day you'd like to eat the majority of your calories.

Hypothetically speaking let's say your macros are 140g protein, 60g fat, and 200g carbs. You can split your macros like this (or any other way):

Two meals a day (Intermittent Fasting)

2PM – 50g protein, 30g fat, 100g carbs
8PM – 100g protein, 30g fat, 70g carbs
Three meals a day

Breakfast – 20g protein, 20g fat, 70g carbs
Lunch – 70g protein, 20g fat, 40g carbs
Dinner – 40g protein, 20g fat, 90g carbs

Three meals a day
1-2PM – 40g protein, 20g fat, 70g carbs
5PM – 60g protein, 30g fat, 40g carbs
8PM – 60g protein, 20g fat, 70g carbs

Four meals a day
Breakfast – 40g protein, 20g fat, 30g carbs
Lunch – 50g protein, 10g fat, 50g carbs
Snack – 30g protein, 20g fat, 20g carbs
Dinner – 40g protein, 15g fat, 80g carbs

Selecting a source for protein and starchy carbs

This is the part where we select the foods that'll make the base of your diet.
As for myself i tend to eat the same foods every day, since i enjoy them. Barely any time is spent
cooking and If they start to get boring, i try some different recipes with them..

My personal choice of foods for each day where.:
Lean protein – chicken, beef, eggs and cheese of the low-fat variety
Starchy carbs – potatoes, whole wheat bread, grain and rice , and cereal
Fruits and Veggies – Too many too name but usually some celery and lettuce and so on.

Fats – Normally my fats can be gained from meat and eggs but for cooking i used both olive oil an and butter depending on the recipe im making.

It's up to you now to choose a viable source of nutrients. Select a couple of sources for protein and carbs that you highly enjoy and eat them during everyday life.

Each meal a day should have the same macronutrients.

If you're planning to eat a total of three meals a day you should come up with at least 3 or 4 options for the first meal, 3 or 4 options for lunch and dinner.

This way you can choose each meal of the day from the options you created before. Because each meal contains similar number of calories and macros you have the option to select a different
option for each meal and easily create countless variety of meals.

Here are some examples for you to better understand:

First Meal.

Serving of meat and vegetables

250g chicken breast – 57.72g protein, 4g fat, 250kcal

300-500g vegetables (such as broccoli and lettuce, etc) – 30g carbs, 150kcal
Two slices of bread – 25.3g, 150 kcal
10g oil – 10g fats, 90 kcal
Total: 50g protein, 14g fats, 60g carbs, 640 kcal

Some tuna, bread and vegetables.
7.23g large can of tuna (the ones without any oil) – 42g protein, 190 kcal
3 slices of bread – 44g carbs, 230 kcal
400-400g vegetables – 20g carbs, 110 kcal
10g oil – 10g fats, 90 kcal
Total: 50g protein, 10g fats, 72g carbs, 630 kcal

Second Meal.

Fruit and Cottage Cheese.
low fat cottage cheese – 50g protein 2.5gfat, 4g carbs
berries – 15g carbs, 70 kcal
2 apple – 20g carbs, 144 kcal
Total: 12g protein, 7g fat, 35g carbs, 460 kcal

Protein Bars and Fruit.

100g protein bar – 42g protein, 16g fat, 40g carbs, 380 kcal
1 apple – 20g carbs, 80 kcal
Total: 42g protein, 16g fat, 60g carbs, 460 kca

As you can read for yourself, this is how a person's meal plan might look like. Now they have a variety of choices on what they can eat every day. This week they might chose the first meal for the week or the second meal for the choice of the week. A variety of options can be chosen depending on how far you plan add into your meal plan.

Whenever you get bored with any of the options available to you, then creating more meal plans is a viable options to further continue your goals. So don't be afraid to spice things up a bit.

Chapter 9: Conclusion

If you've successfully read all the way to this part then i would like to both formally thank you and congratulate you on all of your hard work. This shows the kind of dedication required for people willing to put in the effort necessary to reach your goals. Great job!

Using the information available in this short guide can create a fantastic nutrition plan for fat loss, muscle growth or maintenance. As a matter in fact, I'd say you now know more practical information about nutrition than the majority of the population in this world.

Receiving your daily intake for nutrition is quite simple as long as you follow and remember the basic behind it. There's no point in wasting time with supplements, herbs , exotic extracts and other things like that. If you want to succeed in the art of nutrition, then you must master the basics. Apply the information in this guide and I'm sure you'll reach any goal you set yourself up for.

For more resources on nutrition you can check out blog.nutritionhacks.io

If you're looking for an extremely personalized meal planning service for any type of diet and health goals check out - nutritionhacks.io

Made in the USA
Middletown, DE
30 September 2023

39740601R10021